The Kids' Career Library™

# A Day in the Life of a
# **Nurse**

Liza N. Burby

The Rosen Publishing Group's
PowerKids Press™
New York

Thanks to Teresita Gaceta, R.N., of the Dolan Family Health Center in Greenlawn, Theresa Jacob-Ellis, and Jean Bladykas of the North Shore Health System for their help with this book.

Published in 1999 by The Rosen Publishing Group, Inc.
29 East 21st Street, New York, NY 10010

First Edition

Book Design: Erin McKenna

Photo Illustrations: All photo illustrations by Ethan Zindler.

Burby, Liza N.
    A day in the life of a nurse / Liza N. Burby; [photo illustrations, Ethan Zindler]. — 1st ed.
        p.  cm.—(The kids' career library)
    Includes index.
    Summary: Describes the varied tasks and responsibilities of a nurse in an obstetrician's office.
    ISBN 0-8239-5302-5
    1. Nursing—Vocational guidance—Juvenile literature. 2. Nurses—Juvenile literature. [1. Nurses.
    2. Occupations.]
    I. Zindler, Ethan. ill. II. Title. III. Series.
RT82.B794 1998
610.73'06'9—dc21

                                                                 98-7544
                                                                  CIP
                                                                    AC

# Contents

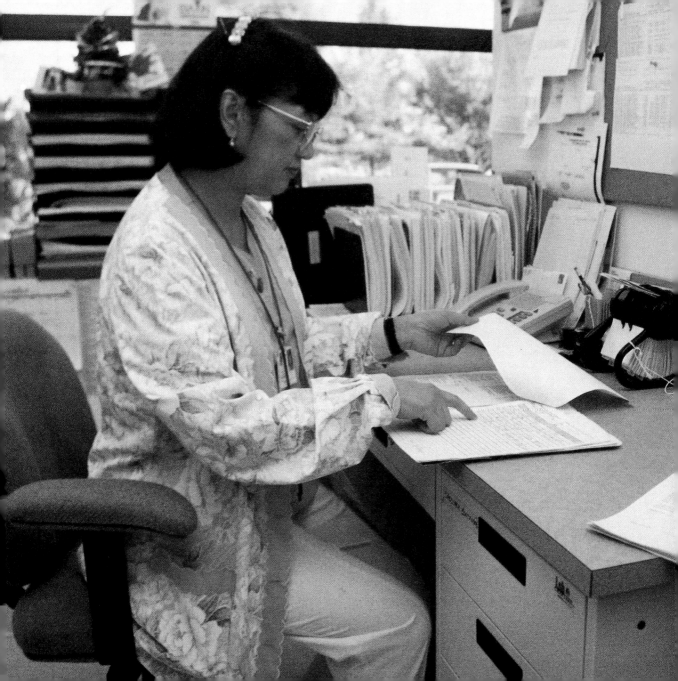

# Running All Day

Teresita Gaceta is a nurse. She works at a family medical center. Her job is to help the **obstetricians** (ob-stuh-TRIH-shunz). These are doctors who take care of women who are **pregnant** (PREG-nunt). Each day Teresita comes to work in her **uniform** (YOO-nih-form). She wears white pants and a bright pink shirt. She believes the pink shirt makes **patients** (PAY-shunts) feel calm. Teresita starts her day by looking at a **schedule** (SKEH-jool). Today, there are women coming to see the doctor almost every five minutes. Teresita will be running around all day!

◀ Teresita must check her schedule every morning so that she knows what her day will be like.

# Pulling Charts

First, Teresita washes her hands. It's important to protect the patients from **germs** (JERMZ). Then she pulls out the **chart** (CHART) for each of the patients she will help today. Some of the women are visiting for the first time. Many will need special tests to make sure that they and their babies are doing well. Teresita prepares the papers that patients will need when they go to a **laboratory** (LA-bruh-tor-ee) for tests. Other women will be having their babies very soon and only need a **checkup** (CHEK-up).

Each patient has a chart that tells Teresita and the doctors about her medical history. ▶

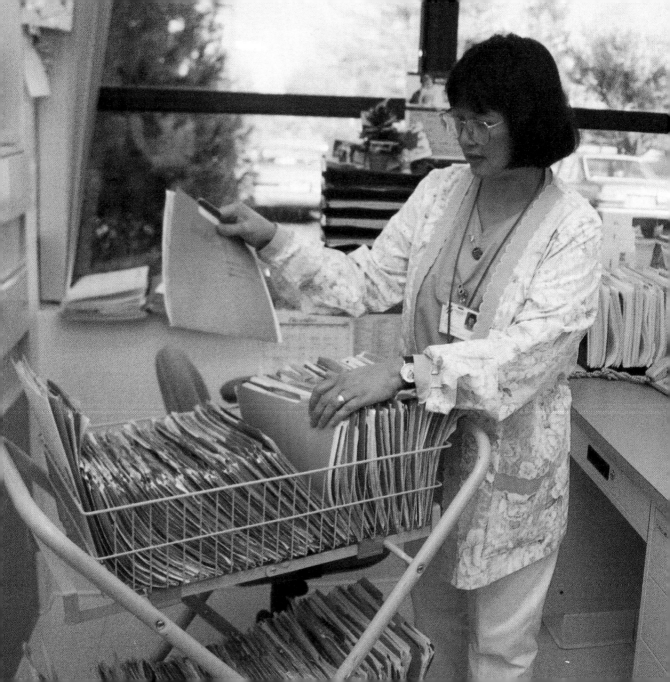

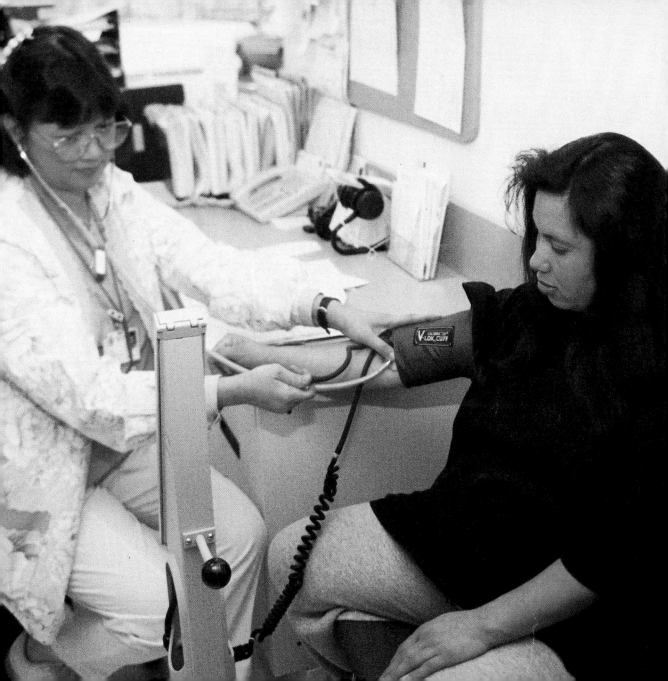

# You Can Come in Now

When the doctor is ready to see the first patient, Teresita goes to the waiting room. "Sylvia, you can come in now," Teresita says. In her office, Teresita does a medical **interview** (IN-tur-vyoo). "Do you have any problems like headaches?" she asks. Sylvia shakes her head no. Teresita listens carefully to Sylvia's heartbeat with a **stethoscope** (STETH-uh-skohp). She checks Sylvia's **blood pressure** (BLUD PREH-shur). Then Teresita weighs Sylvia. Sylvia has gained two pounds since her last visit. That means her baby is growing!

◄ Part of Teresita's job is checking each patient's blood pressure.

9

# Womp! Womp! Womp!

Next, Teresita takes Sylvia to an **examination** (eg-ZA-mih-NAY-shun) room. She asks Sylvia to lie down on the examination table. Teresita makes sure Sylvia is comfortable. Then she asks, "Do you want to hear the baby's heartbeat now?" Sylvia nods. Teresita uses a **Doppler** (DAH-plur). It looks like a funny **microphone** (MY-kruh-fohn). She places it on Sylvia's belly. Suddenly they are able to hear the baby's heartbeat. Womp! Womp! Womp! It is loud and strong. Teresita smiles and says, "That's the nicest sound."

Using just this small Doppler, Teresita is able to ▶ listen to an unborn baby's heartbeat.

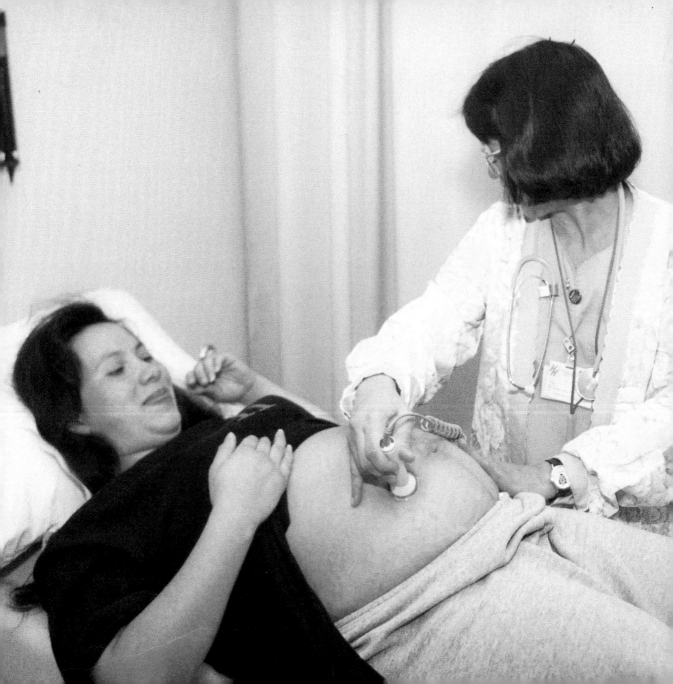

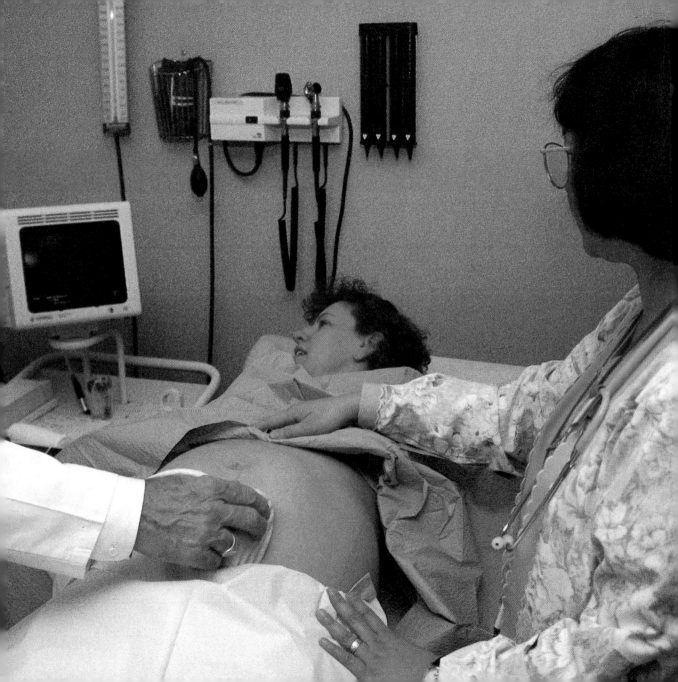

# Helping the Doctor

Next, patients see the doctor. Teresita helps the doctor while he examines each patient. One woman is getting a **sonogram** (SAH-nuh-gram). A sonogram lets the doctor see how a baby looks inside its mother's belly. Teresita's job is to make sure the patient is comfortable. She also gets the doctor whatever he needs to examine the patient. This woman's baby looks healthy. Teresita makes another **appointment** (uh-POYNT-ment) for her. The woman will come back for another checkup in two weeks.

◄ A doctor can sometimes tell if a baby is a boy or a girl from looking at a sonogram.

# Meeting the Babies

Patients also come to the medical center after they have their babies. One mother has a six-week-old baby girl. The mother's back is hurting, and she wants the doctor to check it. Teresita interviews her first. Then the doctor examines the mother. "You will be fine," he tells her. Teresita loves to meet all the new babies. "Look at all your hair," she says to this bright-eyed baby. The baby's mother is proud. Teresita says that one of her favorite things about her job is seeing happy parents after their babies are born.

Teresita enjoys meeting the babies that she ▶ helped care for before they were born.

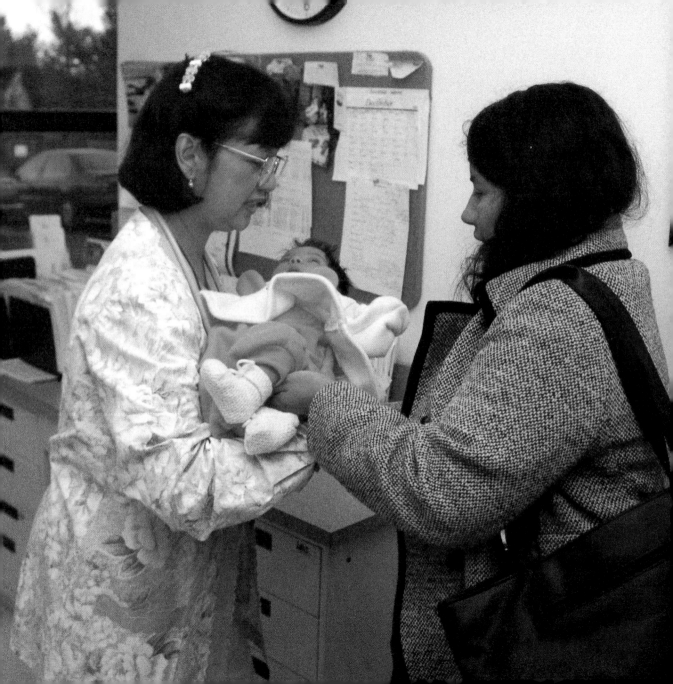

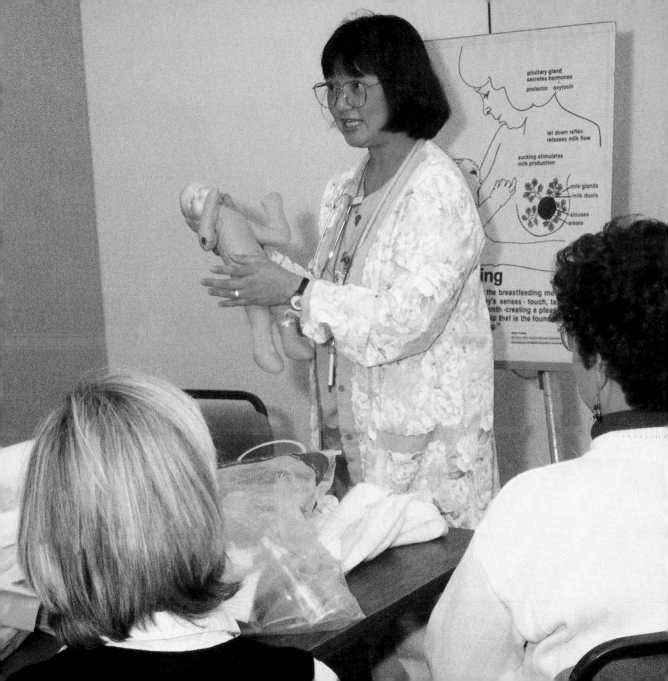

# Teaching Patients

There's a lot to learn about caring for a new baby. Teresita helps new parents by teaching baby-care classes. She answers any questions that parents may have. Teresita shows them how to wash a baby by using a doll. A doll is much easier to bathe than a baby. By watching Teresita, parents learn the proper way to hold a baby. Teresita also shows them how to wrap a baby in a blanket. "New parents are very nervous about doing a good job," she says. Teresita makes the job look easy!

◀ Teresita knows a lot about caring for babies, and she enjoys teaching people everything she knows.

# Never a Rest

Many days, Teresita is too busy to sit down to eat lunch. Sometimes there are **emergencies** (ee-MUR-jen-seez). When she does get a chance to relax, Teresita often spends her time reading nursing magazines. She says that nursing changes all the time as people learn better ways to care for patients. To be the best nurse she can be, Teresita has to learn the newest information. She reads a lot. Teresita studied nursing for four years at college. But she still needs to take classes every three years so that she knows the newest ways to care for patients.

While Teresita eats lunch, she reads the latest nursing magazines to help her be the best nurse she can be. ▶

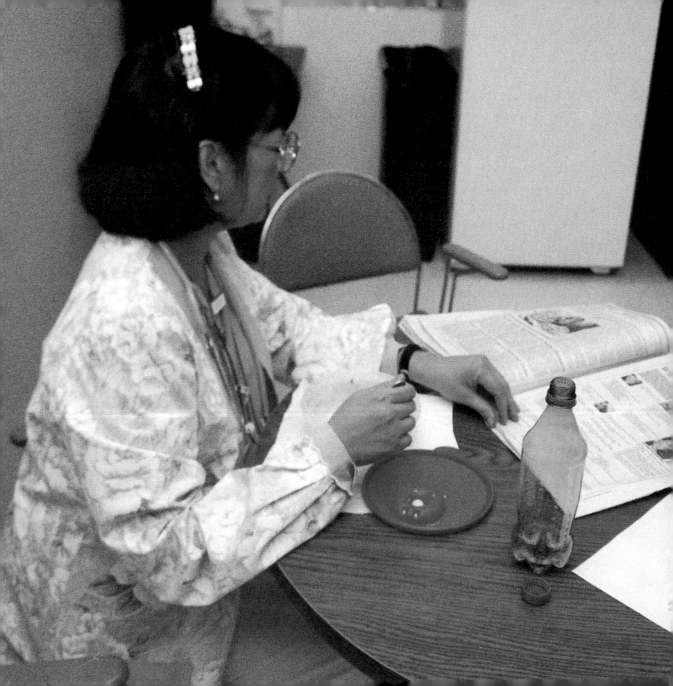

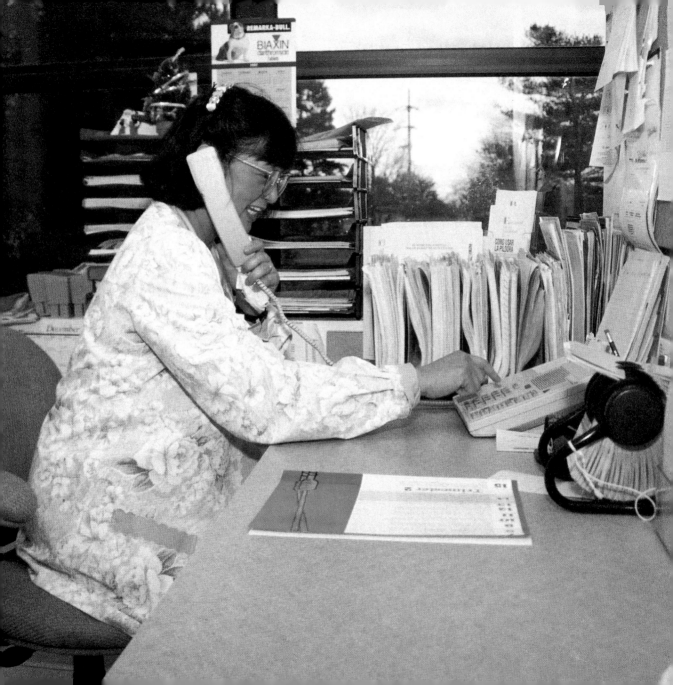

# The End of the Day

Before Teresita's day is over, she must prepare the examination rooms for the next day. Then she calls patients who missed their appointments to make sure they are okay. Teresita prepares charts for tomorrow's patients. She also makes calls to the laboratory to see if a patient's test **results** (ruh-ZULTZ) are ready. She calls the **pharmacy** (FAR-muh-see) to order medicine for a patient. Sometimes there are so many things to do that Teresita must stay at work very late.

◀ Even after all the patients have been seen, Teresita still has lots of work to do.

# This Nurse Loves Her Job

Before she leaves for the day, Teresita looks at all the baby pictures hanging on a wall in her office. These are the babies of her patients. New parents send the pictures to Teresita along with notes thanking her for her help and kindness. Teresita says getting to know patients and their babies is what she loves most about her job. She became a nurse because she wanted to help people. Teresita tries to make her patients feel like they are getting the best care. Tomorrow there will be more patients to care for. Teresita is very happy about that.

# Glossary

**appointment** (uh-POYNT-ment)  A time someone must do something.

**blood pressure** (BLUD PREH-shur)  The pressure created by your heart pumping blood through your body.

**chart** (CHART)  A sheet of paper that lists a patient's medical history.

**checkup** (CHEK-up)  A regular visit to a doctor's office.

**Doppler** (DAH-plur)  A tool used to measure sound waves.

**emergency** (ee-MUR-jen-see)  A sudden need for quick action.

**examination** (eg-ZA-mih-NAY-shun)  When a doctor looks at you carefully.

**germ** (JERM)  A tiny living thing that can cause sickness and infection.

**interview** (IN-tur-vyoo)  To ask someone questions about something.

**laboratory** (LA-bruh-tor-ee)  A room where scientists perform tests.

**microphone** (MY-kruh-fohn)  A device that picks up sounds.

**obstetrician** (ob-stuh-TRIH-shun)  A doctor who treats pregnant women.

**patient** (PAY-shunt)  A person who is being treated by a doctor.

**pharmacy** (FAR-muh-see)  A place where medicine is sold.

**pregnant** (PREG-nunt)  When a woman is going to have a baby.

**result** (ruh-ZULT)  The information that a medical test shows.

**schedule** (SKEH-jool)  A plan of what one has to do at certain times.

**sonogram** (SAH-nuh-gram)  An image produced using sound waves that lets a doctor see a baby while it is growing inside its mother.

**stethoscope** (STETH-uh-skohp)  A tool to listen to someone's heartbeat.

**uniform** (YOO-nih-form)  Special clothes worn for a job.

# Index